To Jackie
With best wishes for a happy,
healthful long life
Zilpha Main

REACHING NINETY -

MY WAY

Good Health and Long Life Can Be Yours, Too

by   Zilpha Pallister Main

Other books by Zilpha Main

COME TRAVEL ALONG TO SOUTH AMERICA AND
TO PANAMA

COME TRAVEL ALONG MOSTLY THROUGH AFRICA
AND THE MIDDLE EAST

COME TRAVEL ALONG AROUND THE WORLD

First edition. Printed in the United States of America

Library of Congress Card Catalog Number 84-90575
ISBN 09601584-5-6 Hardcover, 09601584-6-4 Paperback

Published by Zilpha Main, 2701 Wilshire Blvd., #809
    Los Angeles, CA 90057

In loving memory of my mother
and her devotion to my welfare.

She would have made good use of today's
greater knowledge about nutrition.

FOREWORD

By

Keith E. Kenyon, M.D.

When one considers that this book has been written by a lady who no longer is an octogenarian, its clarity and good sense are remarkable.

Since she has proven by her own longevity that her ideas on nutrition and taking care of herself have been beneficial to her, it would be wise to heed her suggestions.

The scientific aspects of the book are discussed in an easy to understand, clear-cut manner that can make the novice reader much more knowledgeable and conversant.

Moreover, it can be read at one sitting, and it is so easy to comprehend that it reads like a novel.

I salute this exceptional lady and hope that many of her readers will emulate her. If people take care of themselves nutritionally, they can extend their life span by many years.

ACKNOWLEDGEMENTS

Credit and my sincere appreciation for the title of this book goes to Irwin Zucker, founder and president of Promotion in Motion. From the beginning I had thought "Come Travel Along to Fourscore and Ten" would be a rather clever title, but when I told Irwin Zucker that I was not entirely satisfied with it, he suggested exactly what I can't help wishing I had thought of. It is so apt and also brief and catchy. All the rest of the words are mine except, of course, the many quotations. I am grateful to their authors, too.

Then my heartfelt thanks goes to my cousin, Dr. Paul E. Hadley, former vice-president in charge of academic affairs, University of Southern California, for his two readings of this book. My appreciation is not so much for his noting a few misspellings that would have been quite embarrassing, but rather for marking some passages "not clear" and especially for answering all the questions I raised in the margins. Having someone to turn to, even with little problems, is truly a blessing.

I would also thank Charles Crowder, writer and editor, for his reading of the manuscript and his encouragement.

And of course I feel honored as well as grateful to have Keith E. Kenyon, M.D., write an introduction.

PREFACE

Though I invite you to *Come travel along to fourscore and ten* and though I make a few suggestions, I'll not really tell you how to do it. No, just how I've done it. Thought you'd be interested. I'm not even going to tell you how I got over this and that, for I haven't yet had this and that.

But I am curious, and I've wondered about many things. How come I have reached this age? How well do I have things under control? How tell if one is eating right? Should I take vitamins, eat meat, have desserts? What are the basics of nutrition? How well is the body equipped to look after itself? How can I help?

Such are the things I've wondered about and set out to investigate. I've found it a fascinating story. True, I got in deeper than I expected, but I have things in better perspective. I hope you'll feel the same way.

But remember I'm not a nutritionist, just a curious oldster.

Zilpha Main

CONTENTS

ON GROWING OLD (ER)

Everything is farther away now than it used to be; it is twice as far to the corner, and they have added a hill. I have given up running for the bus. It leaves faster than it used to. And it seems to me they are making stairs steeper than in the old days.

Have you noticed the smaller print they are using in the newspaper? And there is no use asking people to read aloud . . . everyone speaks in such a low voice. . . . I ran into an old classmate the other day, and she had aged so much I didn't even recognize her.

I got to thinking about the poor thing this morning while I was combing my hair. And in so doing, I glanced at my reflection. You know, they don't even make mirrors like they used to, either.

Author Unknown

From Mercury Savings
Huntington Beach, CA

PART I

LOOKING AT MY GUIDELINES

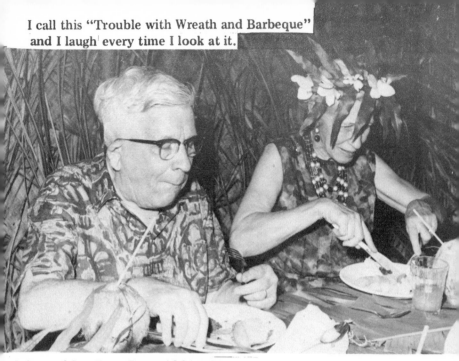

John and I at Bora Bora, 1964, when I was 70

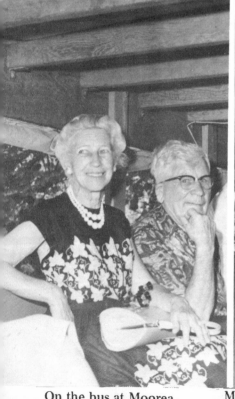

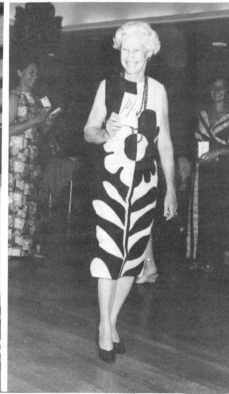

On the bus at Moorea.

Modeling my Tahitian dress on the *Mor*

Prepare

When I say, "Come travel along to fourscore and ten," it can be of course to more than 90 years, but that is all I can speak of with authority at this point, for I was not born until July 10, 1894. (Actually I'm fudging by three months.) On second thought, according to the anti-abortionists I should add nine months to my birth date, which would make me already 90. Now ordinarily one would not want to add nine months to those already galloping years. But who knows, maybe we'll be doing it some day!

Be that as it may, any worthwhile wisdom my years have given me on the matter of adding to the traditional *three*score and ten is a recent acquisition. In fact I am only now think-about it, and do you know, the first pearl that comes to mind is that one should start early preparing for old age. I did. Why, for 30 years I've been carrying a little bottle of nitro-glycerin in my purse—right after I had my first light heart attack in the night. Now, of course, I've never had one in the daytime.

Still I maintain it's good sense to look ahead and to plan for old age. One wants to get all he can out of his future. So I did not wait for 65 to take my social security, oh, no, I might not make that, I thought. So I took mine at age 62. And after I was widowed in '69 at age 75, I was so anxious to leave things in proper shape that I sold our home for $25,000 less than the buyer sold it for a few years later.

Why, I so believe in being prepared that for the last ten years I've had a list made of those to be notified, for I surely wouldn't want folks to be sending me Christmas cards if I were no longer here to receive them.

Yes, start early, be prepared. That's my rule Number One. Must be it's good, for I've reached 89, or 90, as you wish.

Search for an Ancestor or Other Encouragement

Now, of course, there are other, more important ways that I prepared for a long life. Take the matter of ancestors. My grandfathers lived to be 87 and 88, and I had a great-great-grandmother who made it to 87. She was my model, for the rest of the women didn't do so well, my mother dying at 71 and her mother at 44 (my other grandmother reached 71 and my father 80). So it was Great-great-grandmother Deborah Shaw Gibbs who was my inspiration. If she could make it, why couldn't I? Of course, she is down the line quite a way, having been born in 1786, but one can't be too fussy about ancestors. Take them where you find them, I say. So when I passed her age, I turned to my grandfathers, but now I'm without antecedent. Must be there is something else.

In my childhood my mother was careful about what I ate. There weren't any "junk" foods around. No, the fare at our house was plain. It included grits—coarsely ground grain, wheat, I think—vegetables from our city-lot garden, a barrel of apples every fall from my aunt's farm; and for crackers we had arrowroot biscuits, not dainty arrowroot wafers such as you buy in a fancy little box today. No, they were a half inch thick, round, maybe two inches across, scalloped, curved on the bottom (we played they were boats), and they came in a big bag that my mother picked up at the factory. Another thing that marked my childhood was that I usually spent a month on a farm in the summer.

I still think food is terribly important, and I'll give you some of my secrets later. You'll give more thought to them if we first consider aging as the problem that it surely is.

Recognize the Changes

The worst part about aging is that it has only one ending. Still most of us would agree with Jean Abernethy when she says, "I don't mind going, not a mite, but I hate going in this dilapidated condition." (*Old Is Not a Four Letter Word*, 1975, p. 135) Yes, it is typical of old age that it usually brings poorer eyesight, poorer hearing, a diminished sense of taste and smell, and faulty balance. It also brings wrinkles, stiff joints, and impaired memory, circulation, and respiration. Then, too, along with less resilience, there is increased vulnerability to disease. In short, old age is generally marked by waning energy and declining function.

Of themselves these changes in capability cause stress. Then there are the stresses that come from outside oneself. With family grown and retirement, there is apt to creep in a feeling that one is no longer a needed part of society. With further aging comes also the loss of friends. They die, move away to be near family or to a nursing home, and others change mentally. Social reciprocity becomes a burden.

The loss of work-and-social status is particularly hard to bear; it is so much a part of us. Its loss tends to make the old shrink into themselves, and they get dropped by this one, treated condescendingly by that one. Here's a comical instance that actually happened. My friend in a wheelchair was left inside a store entrance while her daughter made a purchase not far away. But she was gone long enough for a couple to stop, make a friendly remark, and—give my friend two quarters.

These changes in capability and the resulting decrease in standing are usually spread over a considerable time span, so that as long as old people feel only minor aches and pains and can function, they are apt to say they feel no different. Even when they sense a difference, it is usually only in degree.

As a friend in her 80's used to say, "I feel as good as ever," and then she would playfully add, "for five minutes."

Another friend in his 80's writes, "When morning comes I feel I could turn the earth over, but by noon I run out of steam." Yes, the old usually have the same feelings and desires as always; it's their energies that wane distressingly.

Those were the fortunate old. Now consider the old in nursing homes. I had a friend who had stayed in two of them. She said that 90 percent of those at the first place were addlebrained. To visit such a place must make one ask, "What can I do to keep out of here?" So let's see what we can do to win at "the aging game." (title of book by Barbara Anderson, 1979)

Get Involved

As I have already said, start early. It is easy in one's 60's, say on retirement. Like as not, you are right off asked to do some sort of volunteer work, but if you don't get asked, look around to see what sort of volunteer work you would best like to do. I chose to be a volunteer for the Los Angeles World Affairs Council. For many years—until I was 80 and my car's interior needed repair—I drove foreign guests of the State Department to appointments, sightseeing, and while my husband was living, we often entertained them in our home.

Any kind of volunteer work helps one to feel useful, even needed, and most likely increases one's stature. In fact, many human betterment projects have been started by older people. The point, I think, is to get involved in the on-going life around us. That is probably the easiest way to adjust to life's fourth season.

Hobbies broaden one's outlook, tend to make one more interesting, and usually give a measure of group activity, as in garden clubs, gem clubs, church clubs. Genealogy may seem to offer little socializing, but it leads to correspondence, sometimes to family gatherings, and occasionally brings surprises. I had a childhood friend who later married a Dr. Samuel Orton. Both names were common in my family history. A little search showed that sure enough we had a common ancestor.

Tracing one's ancestors shows so many roots that it can be an ongoing pursuit. Moreover, it will likely enrich many present and future lives.

Games get us with people and likely improve our skills. Then, too, they temporarily relieve the stresses of life. I find that bridge, played with different groups, is not only good for sociability, but also for sharpening attention, memory, and the thinking process. Yet for me it seems a relaxant, for it is an absorbing change.

Dancing, too, is good, not only for social contact, but also for exercise, especially so in square dancing. Some can continue in the more active sports; others can go fishing for their relaxation.

No question about it, one needs a measure of recreation, but just as surely one needs something more, a sense of progress. Perhaps for the first time in life you now have time to get better informed on the important happenings of the times. My, what an age we are privileged to live in! And there is more to it than the satisfaction of being in on things. The bonus is that you have more to talk about than your health and your reminiscences, and you become a more interesting person, cease to be considered old, and you have grown in stature.

Plan Your Future

Studying some subject that one finds really interesting seems to give purpose to life. So look over the curriculum offered at your level of schooling, or at least pursue your interest in the library. Just on the matter of aging, our library has about six inches of cards.

As one title says, *Everybody's Studying Us* (by Balbal and Paull). Often it is thoroughly, as in Dr. Olga Knoff's *Successful Aging*, and also intriguingly, as in *No More Dying* by Joel Kurtzman and Phillip Gordon. If one book leads to another, most likely you are growing. And surely that is what it is all about.

All these things—volunteer work, hobbies, studying, and various other ongoing pursuits—bring satisfaction and happiness. Also they challenge age and delay and weaken its thrust.

Moreover, they can be pursued to the extent that one can do so with pleasure. Sooner or later we do have to fit our little world to our capabilities, give up some responsibilities, and make fewer demands on ourselves.

So again I say, Start early, be prepared. Plan your future rather than leaving it to others. I've tried. For seven years I've been in this apartment, where *when* I need it I can get help to clean, to get groceries, etc. The grocery is only a block away, and there are two restaurants within a block. The bus stop is here. There is desk service, and my apartment has a beautiful view.

Maybe you would prefer a retirement home. Do look into them while you are able. Or would you want to share your home or share someone else's. In either of these cases you should read Barbara Stanford's *Long Life and Happiness*, 1983.

Exercise, Even If You Don't Feel Like It

People sometimes ask me, "Where do you get all your energy?" For on occasion my calendar shows engagements eight days straight; sometimes I have luncheon and dinner engagements the same day. I drive the freeways without strain, do my own cleaning, get my meals, and lug in groceries, though that is not with ease. I weigh about the same as when I was married (I'm not saying anything about looks); my fingernails are the same size; I have only two small brown spots; I don't have headaches, stomach aches, back aches, or joint aches; I carry a cup without tremor; and I get up from the floor without too much trouble. Keeping mobile is something I feel strongly about, for it seems to me it is the sine qua non for independence. I hope I'm exercising enough to keep out of a wheelchair.

Actually I don't exercise enough, though I thoroughly believe in its benefits. My rationalization is that I belong to the cat family. Cats don't run their legs off as dogs do, yet how easily and fast they can run when there is need. So I say, Let the dog family run, I'll do as the cats do—I'll stretch and turn. Now of course if you belong to the dog family, by all means jog or whatever.

I admit I feel better the days I'm active, and I regularly pay token homage to the Exercise god. On waking in the morning I just lie in bed and stretch all over—like a cat, and I get up feeling fine. Another concession I make to Exercise is that I run the 25 feet that my apartment allows. I've read that the blood circulates 55 feet per minute when the body is at rest, but up to 450 feet per minute with vigorous exercise. That way it carries off a lot of toxins. So I run until I get tired, which isn't very long. The days I'm just reading and writing I aim to do this hourly, but I never do.

I get so absorbed in my work that I forget. Yet I cannot complain about my memory. I am rarely bothered about remembering where I put things, for I take pains to note where I lay them. But now to the matter of exercise.

Here's a Short Exercise Regimen

Besides stretching and spurt running, it's also been my custom to lie on the floor and raise my feet a few times (knees straight), then bicycle a bit. I've been doing that for some time. Recently I've added Linda Clark's Five Tibetan Rites as given in her *Rejuvenation Programme* (1980). Here's my abbreviated version:

1. With arms outstretched at the sides make complete turns clockwise until slightly dizzy.
2. Lie on your back and raise your legs as far as you can, keeping knees straight.
3. Sit on the floor. Put palms on the floor a bit back. Bend knees. Then with soles on the floor raise your body to make a table.
4. Kneel on the floor with hands on thighs. Lean as far forward as you can, then as far back as you can, letting head fall back.
5. Kneel and put palms on the floor, then straighten your knees to raise your hips as high as you can, letting head hang down. Next let the body sag, but with head held up.

These exercises are to be practiced once each, three times a day to begin with, working up to 21 times a day. I aim to do them four or five times each and two to four times a day.

One day I found myself looking around for something to get hold of to help me get up. Here's what I found to avoid that: From a kneeling position I raised my right knee, put my right hand on it, and with the help of a push from the floor with my left hand, I was up without trouble. Maybe I've invented an exercise. Anyhow, if I have need, I do it two or three times.

After all, the important thing about any exercise is that it make use of the muscles that need strengthening. So, as part of Exercise 2, I pull my bent knees toward my chest with my hands, then spread them apart. Hope this keeps me able to put on my stockings. Had a friend who couldn't.

Feet, Too, Need Exercise

My running is always without shoes. In fact, I have not
worn shoes in the house for many years, not since we visited
Japan. I wear "peds." It is better for the feet to get all the
movement possible. For, mind you, each foot has 28 bones,
20 muscles, and 112 ligaments, which tie the bones together,
besides the networks of bloodvessels and nerves. Then there
are the tendons that attach the muscles to the bones.

Just standing, the weight of the whole body is transmitted
from the ankle bones to the heel bones to the ground, the
other structures giving balance. But when walking the entire
foot is in action, and as podiatrist Dr. Morton Walker points
out, "The feet of a man who weighs one hundred and sixty-
five pounds lift and carry—in terms of his personal weight
only—about sixteen hundred tons every day." (*Your Guide
to Foot Health*, 1964, p. 29)

Even when sitting at my desk I stretch my feet and legs.
Dr. Walker gives nine specific exercises for the feet, pp. 7-12.
I'd like to describe one, for it is designed "to bring into use
every muscle of balance." It consists of crossing the legs while
standing, placing the feet parallel and slightly apart. After
holding that position a minute or so, reverse, again keeping
the weight evenly distributed. Start with hands on chair back.

I usually get up easily from an 18-inch chair, but it helps
if one puts one foot back of the chair edge and leans forward
so that the weight of the body is equally distributed.

What I do not find easy is lugging in groceries, though with
a single sack it does help some if I carry the sack in front
with both arms supporting the load. Still there are the steps,
where in addition to lifting my body there are the heavy bags.

Then there are the doors to be opened. That's when I am
thankful for the plastic bags that can be set down and picked
up, for I have doors to: the lobby, the hall, the elevator (two
entering and two leaving), and my apartment. By then I am
thinking: "If only I didn't have to eat!" What a saving that
would be of time, energy—and money!

Food Poses Other Questions

On the other hand, eating is such a wonderful and pleasant way to get energy. After enjoying the flavor of our food, we merely have to chew and swallow it. Then our built-in processing plant uses it to activate the digestive system, the glands, muscles, nerves, and the brain. My, how marvelously we are made, how wonderfully equipped! And all we have to do is fuel the processing plant. In short, just give the body the nourishment it needs.

Ah; there's the rub. Much has been written about how to stay in the pink of health, but right off we find three classes of diet: vegetarian, ovo-lacto, and mixed. The difference is based on protein, not the need for it, but the amount and source. Both the vegetarian and the egg-milk diets call for less protein than the Food and Nutrition Board of the National Research Council proposes, and so do the diets of some advocates of the mixed diet.

The recommended dietary allowance (RDA) of protein that the Board proposes is one gram of protein daily for each 2.2 pounds of body weight. Figure your proper intake according to your proper weight. For example, my 90 pounds divided by 2.2 gives 41 and one gram each makes 41 grams of protein my needed daily intake. What is yours by this standard?

Now, the protein we eat is broken down into 22 amino acids, the so-called building blocks of body protein. Of these 22 amino acids, eight are essential for adults, meaning we have to furnish them in our diet. The body can synthesize the others, provided the essential ones are provided. Some foods contain all eight of the essential amino acids. Others do not. Those that do are called complete.

In the following table of complete protein foods, only those of animal origin have the amino acids in adequate and balanced amounts. However, other foods with protein in them can be combined to do very well, as Frances Moore Lappe shows in *Diet for a Small Planet*. For example, baked beans

and steamed brown bread or beans and rice complement each
other in the essential amino acids.

Complete Protein Foods			
¼ lb. lean meat, fish, or fowl	15-25	mg.	protein
2 oz. American Cheddar cheese	14	"	"
2 large eggs	13	"	"
½ cup cottage cheese	13	"	"
½ cup soybeans (cooked)	10	"	"
1 cup milk	9	"	"
2 tb. soybean flour	8	"	"
¼ cup wheat germ	7	"	"
2 tb. brewer's yeast	8	"	"

Values taken from *Nutrition Almanac*, John D. Kirschmann, Dir., 1979,
pp. 202-26.

The preceding table includes milk, and I would mention
that milk as we generally get it does not stand in unques-
tioned repute. In fact, pasteurization largely destroys its B
vitamins, also A and C, while homogenization so completely
and permanently breaks up the fat particles that the enzyme
xanthine oxidase gets into the blood stream and thus into the
arterial walls and muscles, and so causes atherosclerosis. This
may not be finally proven, but for the last year or so I've
been drinking certified raw milk, which Henry Bieler, M.D.,
so strongly advocates in *Food Is Your Best Medicine*.

Watch Your 40-60 Diet

What I'm eating now may be rather irrelevant, for as Gaye-lord Hauser says, "What you eat between the ages forty and sixty largely determines how you feel, look, and think at seventy and eighty. But it is never too late." (Gaylord Hauser's *New Treasury of Secrets*, 1974, p. 10)

Looking back, I guess we did eat pretty sensibly in that period: for breakfast, fruit juice or fruit, oatmeal or shredded wheat biscuit, a hermit made with nuts, dates, and raisins, and one cup of coffee (mine mostly water); for lunch, a whole-wheat sandwich (egg, fish, or meat), milk or butter-milk, and probably something fresh, at least lettuce; and for dinner, a green salad, meat, fish, or fowl, potato, a vegetable, and dessert, which was most often ice cream and fruit, but for company it might be Dear Abbey's pecan pie, of which she said, "Nothing tops this one." Now I usually don't bother with dessert, but might have a graham cracker.

Being alone the last 15 years, I have given more thought and study to foods, and I credit my good health largely to my diet regimen, especially perhaps to my breakfast mix. The idea of a mix probably came from Adelle Davis's Pep-Up (*Let's Get Well*, 1965, p. 413) and Gladys Lindberg's Seren-ity Cocktail (now in *Take Charge of Your Health*, 1982, p. 152). Linda Clark lists similar ingredients in her *Stay Young Longer*, 1968, p. 211. Then there's Dr. Rinse's recipe (See Morton Walker, *How Not to Have a Heart Attack*, 1980, p. 114), and in *Earl Mindell's Vitamin Bible* that author's mix, p. 245 and 254. These nutrition experts had no age group in mind, but they'd surely agree that those 40-60 should take precautions.

As for my mix, I can hardly say it has scientific research back of it. My, no! It just evolved as I read about this and that and decided I should be sure to get some every day. The easiest way to do that was to put it in my mix.

The Dry Ingredients for My Potpourri

Take brewer's yeast. It's one of the two nutrients that appear to be in everyone's recipe. Must be it's good. In fact, it is called a complete food. It has most of the amino acids of protein (all eight that the body needs to have supplied), 14 minerals, and 17 vitamins. So it is that yeast is called a wonder food.

Lecithin also appears to be in everyone's recipe. Its special virtue is that it dissolves plaques already laid down in the arteries. So it is especially helpful in treating arteriosclerosis. Lecithin, usually obtained from soybeans, is found in every cell, and it is said to be 40 percent of the brain. That's for me.

Soybean flour, like yeast, is called a complete food. Not only are soybeans high in protein, "In addition, soybeans contain vitamins and minerals in a natural relationship that is similar to the human body's needs." (*Nutrition Almanac*, John D. Kirschmann, Dir., 1979, p. 189)

But all of these foods—brewer's yeast, lecithin, and soybean flour—are high in phosphorus, and phosphorus needs calcium to function effectively, in fact, at least as much calcium as phosphorus. Then calcium needs magnesium, roughly half as much magnesium as calcium. So, as Dr. Rosenberg advises in *The Book of Vitamin Therapy*, 1974, p. 117, I added dolomite, which has approximately that ratio. Since dolomite may contain some lead, it may be safer to use calcium lactate or calcium gluconate and magnesium. In any case, one can adjust the magnesium for regularity.

Alfalfa is high in chlorophyll. Says N. W. Walker, D.Sc., "One of the richest chlorophyll foods we have is alfalfa. It is a food that builds up both animals and humans, all things considered, into a healthy, vital, and vigorous old age, and builds up a resistance to infection that is almost phenomenal." (*Fresh Vegetable and Fruit Juices*, 1981, p. 28) Alfalfa is rich in enzymes and vitamins, especially vitamin K, which is antihemorrhaging.

Kelp, too, is loaded with vitamins and minerals. I use only a small amount. It is strong in iodine; in fact, one teaspoon of kelp contains four mg. of iodine, which is the amount that Adelle Davis recommends per day.

Those are the dry ingredients of my breakfast mix. I'll give the amounts after commenting on the liquid ingredients.

The Liquids in My Mix

First comes yogurt. Being a fermented milk, it has all of
the nutrients of milk plus the yogurt bacteria that predigest
its protein, make calcium easier to digest, break down cholesterol, and provide friendly bacteria for the so-called intestinal
flora. Who wouldn't want yogurt every day?

And we need oils, especially the three essential fatty
acids—linoleic, linolenic, and archidonic, which are found
respectively in safflower, soy, and peanut oils. These are
called essential because the body can't make them; however, if it gets the linoleic, then it can make the other two.
These oils are necessary for utilizing cholesterol and saturated
fats. I used to buy these oils separately, then bought a
blend, and now use safflower and sunflower, since I often
use peanut butter and soy products. I now also add codliver
oil. It contains vitamin D, which is needed for calcium to
be utilized. Then, too, fish liver oils are a top source of vitamin A.

Next, my mix gets some black-strap molasses, another
"wonder" food. I think I added it when I read how it cured
the guinea pigs that had been made so arthritic that they
could not right themselves when laid on their sides. No, not
until they had been fed black-strap molasses. And it is also
good for treating anemia.

Then I like fresh pineapple juice, so I add some of that.
It has enzymes and helps digestion. Moreover, it is said that
bromelain, an enzyme in fresh pineapple, acts as a "pipe
cleaner" for blood vessels, and so it helps to prevent arteriosclerosis and heart attack.

My Personal Recipe

This provides enough for four or five days, and of the dry ingredients I make six or seven recipes at a time. With these measurements the dry ingredients can be kept mixed. With larger amounts the lecithin tends to be on top and the dolomite on the bottom.

Dry Ingredients	Liquid Ingredients
2/3 cup lecithin	1 pt. (2 cups) plain yogurt
1/3 " brewer's yeast	1½ tb. safflower oil
1/4 " soy flour	1½ tb. sunflower seed oil
1½ tb. dolomite	1 tb. codliver oil
1 tb. alfalfa powder	1½ tb. black-strap molasses
1 t. powdered kelp	Stir and add
	½ cup pineapple juice

Each day I pour about a half cupful of the liquid mixture in a large cup, add a quarter of a cup of the dry mix, and stir. Then I add some cut-up fruit, say half a peach or apple. That ensures chewing and provides flavor. This mixture is sort of like porridge, though of course it could be diluted with milk or juice. But it is easy to just pour the liquid part, add the dry mix, cut up the fruit, and eat with a spoon. Afterwards it is important to drink a cup of liquid. Of course the amounts of the mix that I use are for my weight. You might want more. And of course, made more liquid, it could be drunk throughout the day. After all, it's just food. Still, in spite of my high regard for this mix, I take it only six mornings a week.

My Diet in General

When I go out I eat and enjoy whatever is served. The only exception is tea, coffee, and alcoholic drinks. I simply never learned to like them, so I take water or for cocktails a soft drink or a juice, if offered. At home I follow a plain, mostly natural foods routine. I either have no dessert or a little fresh fruit, or dried fruit (say, a couple of dates), or a little of the coffeecake I brought home from a meeting. There isn't any natural food I haven't always liked except buttermilk. But my husband liked that, and I learned, though at first I held my nose closed.

Still, I have trouble understanding people not liking this and that, but I put it down as due to individual difference. And I do think each of us has a built-in mentor.

Now, I seldom eat meat, usually having liver, chicken, or fish, especially sardines, or eggs. I aim to have some protein each meal, maybe cottage cheese or *tofu*. I like baked potato, and I'm fond of broccoli. But then I like everything.

The cholesterol scare over eggs failed to recognize that the body makes cholesterol, and an excess can be handled by adding lecithin to emulsify it. In fact, egg yolk itself is a rich source of lecithin. So I have at least four eggs a week, usually more.

When I have company, I often serve a combination vegetable dish of equal amounts of cut-up celery, string beans, zucchini, and in season some jicama. With butter and seasonings added, I think you'll like it, and these three non-starchy vegetables complement each other to rid the body of toxins. With parsley added, they are the ingredients for "Dr. Bieler's Broth." (*Food Is Your Best Medicine*, 1966, p. 23) Anyhow here's a dish that helps your guests feel comfortable after your gourmet best.

When fixing that combination for myself, I usually peel the zucchini and cook the peelings with the string beans, eating the peeled zucchini and celery raw.

Something Raw Every Meal

The fact is I try to get something raw every meal. For 900 cats can't be wrong! Some time ago I was impressed with Dr. Francis Pottenger, Jr.'s experiments with all those cats. He fed one half of them raw milk and raw meat and the other half of them, cooked meat and pasteurized and evaporated milk. The first group remained healthy generation after generation, while the second group got less and less healthy.

In fact, when dropped from a certain height, the third generation cats of the second group could not get up. Yet when the third generation of the first group were dropped from the same height, these cats showed the same agility as the first generation.

The explanation is that raw foods have enzymes, which are killed by heating, even by pasteurization, but when raw they set off in the living cell the biochemical processes of life itself.

I also aim to have a glass of raw milk every day, plus the half cup of yogurt at breakfast. I think that is enough milk for me, so I don't use powdered milk.

Raw vegetable and fruit juices stand high in my estimation, still I do not prepare them. And I don't buy as much as I would if they were dated as milk is. As things are, I buy mostly from the factory and so feel surer that I get juice prepared that day. Both carrot juice and the vegetable mix, made of carrot, celery, parsley and spinach juices, are made daily, and pineapple juice three times a week.

Raw juices have only the fiber removed, so the nutrients remain. The vitamins and minerals are absorbed within minutes to serve as coenzymes. The minerals also serve as atomic elements of the body.

Then, too, I take vitamin and mineral supplements and have for some years. Yet I've wondered and wondered how necessary, which ones, what amounts, and so on. But how to find answers to such questions without first considering how the body works?

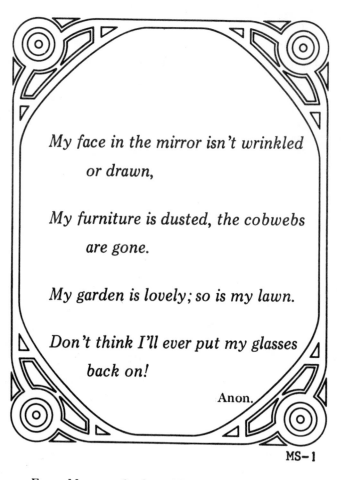

My face in the mirror isn't wrinkled or drawn,

My furniture is dusted, the cobwebs are gone.

My garden is lovely; so is my lawn.

Don't think I'll ever put my glasses back on!

Anon.

MS-1

From Mercury Savings, West Los Angeles, CA

PART II

GETTING DOWN TO BASICS

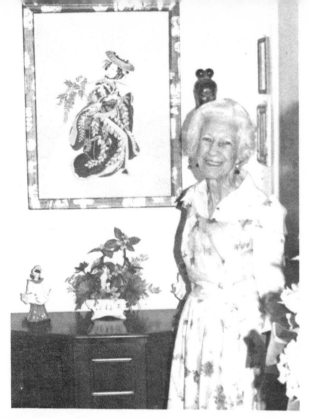

December, 1978, in my apartment, when I was 84

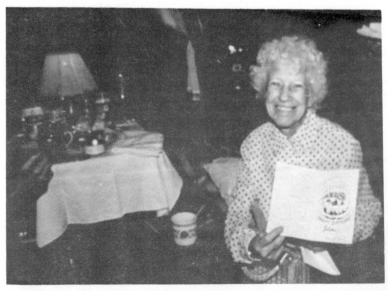

Celebrating my 87th birthday, July, 1981 on the *Central Kingdom Express* in Mongolia

Let's Follow the Food Route

This far I've told you what I've done, not so much to reach four score and ten years, but to do so with good blood pressure (130 over 70), a good blood picture, no getting up nights, taking care of my apartment and food, driving, active in club work, and authoring my fourth book. I've told you the practical things I've learned. I trust you have found it interesting and have profited in some measure.

Now let's see how our processing plant works, what it consists of, what fuel it's getting, and then maybe we'll get a better idea about what we should give it.

Perhaps you already are following a healthful regimen, and this may merely clarify something here and there. For others considerable change may seem called for, and that means that greater understanding is needed. People stop smoking once they are truly convinced that that is the sensible thing to do. And people change eating habits if it makes better sense to do so.

So first let's see what happens to the food we eat. We are so accustomed to eating. (Why, the average person is said to consume half a ton a year.) We're so interested in its taste. Just watch how often food takes over in conversation. And the process of digestion is so automatic and complicated that it is no wonder it gets little attention by the average person. But, oh, how fascinating it is!

In following the food route we'll see what happens at the various stations, we'll consider the motility (the mixing and the transport), the breaking down of food mechanically and chemically so that it can be used, and then we'll note how it is absorbed. Needless to say, this account is over-simplified, but the whole process is fabulous.

The Mouth, Reception Room and Workshop

The tastebuds, located on the upper surface of the tongue, are individually sensitive to sweet, sour, salt, and bitter, and some to more than one. In combination and aided by the olfactory sense, they give us flavor. Chewing allows for more taste and also breaks up the food. Saliva, which is 98-99.5 percent water, moistens the food.

Saliva flows all the time, but the presence of food causes the glands to excrete more. It is estimated as much as 600 ml. per day. With 29.57 ml. per liquid ounce, that means about 20 ounces or 2½ cups per day. And on occasion it can be much more. For example, "Salivary flow increases rapidly when food or substances with a strong sour taste are ingested." (McGraw-Hill Encyclopedia 1977, V. 4, p. 176) The three main pairs of salivary glands are the sublingual under the tongue, the submaxillary under each jaw at the back, and the parotid in front of each ear. The saliva contains mucin, a protein that lubricates, and the enzyme *ptyalin*.

Enzymes are basically protein, and they act as catalysts, that is, they cause a chemical reaction without being changed themselves. (more later) The ptyalin here converts pure starches into dextrin and maltose, which are absorbable. This is significant for being the first chemical reaction and the only absorption in the mouth. It explains why nitroglycerin under the tongue is effective, also the easy absorption of alcohol, not so much in the mouth, for it isn't there long, but it is made ready for absorption.

Right along with chewing and the activity of the salivary glands, the motility of the tongue plays its part. Just for once do take note. You'll surely be impressed with its agility in the chewing process. Then, when the food is ready for swallowing, we use the tongue for forcing it into the pharynx. It is amazing how the nasal valve is closed, but that is automatic.

The esophagus, which is 9-12 inches long, has a valve top and bottom. Its muscles work by peristalsis, that is, by wave-like contraction and relaxation to move the food along.

The Stomach, Storage and Mixing Room

Ordinarily a meal's stay in the stomach is 2-5 hours. Water passes right through. It is interesting that the mucosa lining the stomach is of two kinds: the oxyntic glandular mucosa, which lines the upper part of the stomach, and the pyloric glandular mucosa, which lines the lower part. It is the oxyntic cells that produce Hcl (hydrochloric acid), also pepsinogen and, for the later absorption of B/12, the so-called Intrinsic Factor, a muco-protein enzyme.

The stomach's main business is breaking down protein, mainly with Hcl and pepsin. The Hcl is surprisingly strong, having a pH of 1.0 when fresh and 2.0 when diluted with the gastric contents. *pH* is the symbol for acidity, which is based on a scale of 0-14, water (neutral) being 7. The Hcl rate of secretion reaches its maximum in the second half hour after a meal is begun. Hcl gives to pepsinogen the acid it, too, needs to become effective in breaking down protein. Hcl kills anything live and so prevents bacterial putrefaction. One might wonder about the stomach wall itself, but its secretion of slimy mucin gives it protection. Then, too, it is replaced by new cells every two to three days.

The total amount of acid secreted for a meal is directly proportional to the amount of protein in that meal, so in a largely starchy meal the ptyalin can likely continue its action for some time in the stomach.

As to the secretion in the lower part of the stomach, it contains no Hcl. And whereas the wall of the upper part of the stomach was relatively quiet, the wall of the lower part makes strong peristaltic contractions. The mixing that thus takes place means the end of any salivary ptyalin action on starch and also the thorough mixing of Hcl and pepsin with the food.

In fact, this is where the digestion of protein starts. Here the Hcl and the pepsin begin the breakdown of protein into amino acids. Since older people frequently lack Hcl and pepsin, they often benefit from supplements of these digestants.

Yet Horace Davenport says, "Acid and pepsinogen are not essential for protein digestion." (*A Digest of Digestion*, 1975, p. 51) Indeed, one can do without a stomach, but it sure is good to have.

Fat is broken down to a slight extent by the stomach's secretion of lipase, and sometimes more is regurgitated from the duodenum.

I'm omitting the part the autonomic nervous system plays in all this, but it should be mentioned that fear or rage depresses gastric activity, whereas continued anxiety or hostility causes too much gastric secretion and thereby causes ulcers.

Since the wall of the stomach is highly convoluted, it only makes space as food enters it. It can stretch a lot, even to hold maybe 1½ quarts. Moreover, it has millions of gastric glands, which secrete a pint to a quart of gastric juices for a meal. Amazing, isn't it?

The food is pushed on from the stomach only when it is sufficiently broken down and the duodenum is empty enough to receive it.

The Duodenum, End of the Line
in the Breaking-down Process

The length of the duodenum is only the width of 12 fingers, about 10 or 11 inches. In its wall is a duct called the common bile duct, because it brings bile from the liver or the stored supply in the gallbladder, and just before it enters the duodenum, this duct is joined by the pancreatic duct. The release of secretions from these three (the pancreas, the liver, and the gallbladder) is set off on the arrival of the broken-down food. The secretion of all three is alkaline. So the acidity, which was necessary for pepsin to do its work of breaking down protein in the stomach and to prevent putrefaction of food there, is now turned to alkalinity.

The pancreatic juice contains the enzyme trypsin, which acts on proteins to form amino acids, though some protein, as noted, has already been so changed. Pancreatic juice also contains the enzyme amylase, which changes starch to dextrin and then to maltose. Then, too, the pancreatic juice contains the enzyme lipase, which turns fats to glycerol and fatty acids. Moreover, the bile salts of the pancreatic secretion treble its fat-splitting power. The bile secretion also contains cholesterol; in fact, cholesterol is needed to form bile. And with the bile, lecithin, produced by the liver, likewise enters the duodenum. All three work to emulsify fats.

The motility of the duodenum is seen in both peristalsis and segmentation. The latter means that contractions are spaced uniformly, and they occur as often as 10 times a minute. So by mechanical as well as chemical action, the duodenum delivers the broken-down food in a neutral and equally concentrated state. And mind you, it does all this in just minutes. So now the broken-down food and gastric secretions are in shape for absorption—for use in nourishing the body.

The Jejunum and the Ileum—where you get nourished

Together these two sections of the intestinal tract are about 20 feet long. There's no valve between them, but they differ in that the jejunum has fewer lymph nodules, a thicker membrane, and the villi lining it are larger.

Now the villi (there are some in the duodenum too) are hairlike and only .1-1.5 mm. in length. Always moving, they absorb the nutrients in the chyme, the broken-down food. Unbelievably structured, each villus contains a network of capillaries and a lymphatic vessel. See next page.

It is these tiny villi that absorb the nutrients from the chyme, which, as stated, now has the protein broken down into amino acids, the carbohydrates into glucose, and the fats into glycerol and free fatty acids. By their smooth muscles being shortened and lengthened, the villi move these materials along to the blood and lymph vessels.

The blood vessels carry the amino acids and glucose to the portal vein, then to the liver and general circulation, while lymph vessels carry the glycerol and fatty acids to the main lymphatic trunk, the thoracic duct, and eventually to the right atrium of the heart.

Besides the villi, there are the columnar cells lining the intestinal wall. These also are absorptive. So efficient are the villi and columnar cells that 30-50 percent of the protein is broken down and absorbed within 15 minutes of leaving the stomach. In fact, most of the material passing from the stomach to the end of the ileum requires only 30-90 minutes. Yet the passage through the colon takes roughly one to seven days.

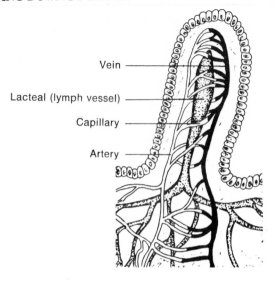

Structure of a villus.

From Louis Levine in *Biology for a Modern Society*,
The C. V. Mosby Co. St. Louis, 1977, p. 106.

The Colon, the System's Draining Plant

The large intestine is about three feet long and has three main sections: the ascending colon, the transverse, and the descending. Its mucosa secretes mucus but no enzymes, yet it has bacteria that produce nicotinic acid and vitamin K. It has no villi, but it absorbs some calcium, magnesium, and iron.

The colon's main function is to absorb water for reuse. What the rectum excretes is dead mucosal cells, indigestible material, but mostly bacteria.

The secretion and absorption story is nicely summed up for us by Dr. Frank L. Eban, "A normal person daily ingests about 3,000 ml. of liquid and food, the gastrointestinal tract adds 8,000 to 14,000 ml. of digestive juices and nearly all are absorbed, so that only 200 gr. of solid is evacuated from the intestinal tract." In *Modern Nutrition in Health and Disease*, edited by R. Goodhart and M. Shils, 6th ed. 1980, p. 35.

The Cell, End of the Nourishment Line

With the nutrients that we ate now in the blood and lymph systems, it is mostly the cells that absorb them. But cells are not just little sponges. They're organized substances, or should I say "bits of life," working constantly to make energy and maintain the body they are in. To get a better idea of how they do this and then to see how we can help, let's consider their structure and how they operate. It is an amazing story and much of it only recently known.

Now the yolk of a chicken's egg is a cell, but human cells are microscopic. The largest is the female's ovum, which is the size of a pinpoint. Yet all cells have a membrane, in which is the protoplasm. It's defined as the chemically active mixture of water, protein, fats, carbohydrates and more that form the living matter in which metabolism, growth, and reproduction are manifest. The cell's protoplasm is a busy place.

Except for red blood cells, all animal cells have a nucleus and within that a nucleosis. That and more had been learned with the light microscope, which magnifies up to 2,000 times. With the development in 1932 of the electron microscope, which uses beams of electrons instead of beams of light, magnifications up to 200,000 times can be obtained.

So now it is known that the outer membrane of a cell is in three layers, two of protein sandwiching one of fat. Then, too, the stringy appearance of the protoplasm has been found to be networks of ducts and various tiny working units. The diagram on page 39 shows these and the other main structures in the cell. Maybe you'd like to read a bit more about some of them.

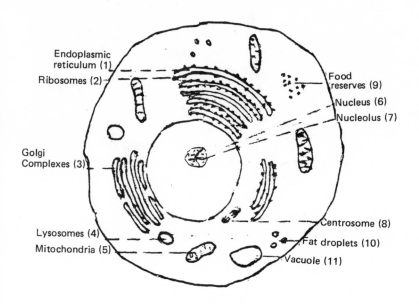

Diagram of a cell

The Cell's Amazing Structures

The *ER* (endoplasmic reticulum) or innerplasmic network (1). This system has rough and smooth membranes. The rough ones form sheets wherein amino acids are synthesized and transported. The smooth ones form tubes wherein is synthesis and transport of carbohydrates and lipids (fats).

Ribosomes, innumerable small granules active in protein synthesis (2). Some ribosomes are attached to the ER, some are not.

Golgi Complexes (3). These are similar to the ER. They consist of hollow stacked discs, and they, too, have to do with the synthesis and transport of protein, but they also handle polysaccharides (sugars).

Lysosomes (4). These are round floating structures, whose function is digestive. They gather around certain materials, including harmful ones, and engulf them.

Mitochondria (5). These are sausage-shaped capsules filled with two-fold membranes—lumps of thread (*mitos*, thread; *chondros*, lump). Mitochondria chemically convert food into energy, which is transported by means of an acid, ATP (axenosine triphosphate). More precisely, mitochondria oxidize carbohydrates, fats, and proteins to release energy, carbon dioxide and water. And mitochondrial contraction is related to respiratory activity. Mitochondria are in every type of cell except red blood cells.

Nucleus (6), without which the cells could not divide. Throughout the nucleus is a protein substance called chromatin. It is both granular and in strands, the latter resembling a network. For cell division the strands, called chromosomes, shorten and thicken, but they have a weak center that breaks. After regrouping they form two cells, each still with 46 chromosomes, the constant number in human cells.

The molecular structure of chromosomes is DNA (deoxyribonucleic acid). It contains the pattern, not only of all body functions but also of hereditary matter. And mind you, DNA is double-stranded with the two strands having many inter-connections. Moreover, it is coiled. So a model looks like a spiraled staircase. I'm putting in this detail for the marvel of it, but it is said, "Damage to DNA is now accepted as a major cause of aging." (Durk Pearson and Sandy Shaw, *Life Extension*, 1981, p. 76) The DNA carries instructions also to the ribosomes, which make protein. To reach outside the nucleus, DNA depends on RNA (ribonucleic acid, its so-called messenger.)

Nucleolus (7), an area of condensed filaments and granules, which are involved in the production of RNA.

Centrosome (8), usually found near the cell's nucleus. This tiny body separates into two parts and attracts the divided chromosomes in cell division.

Food Reserves (9, 10). These consist of small particles and fat droplets.

Vacuole (11), a cavity containing fluid.

Enzymes, Where Vitamins Work

Enzymes are in cells and also in non-cellular material. In the discussion of the digestive tract, mention was made of several enzymes: ptyalin, pepsin, trypsin, amalase, and lipase. Enzymes are complex substances produced in living cells, either wholly or partially protein, that act as catalysts. They speed up reactions without themselves being changed.

Enzymes are generally classed as digestive or metabolic. One readily thinks of the digestive enzymes in the salivary glands, the stomach, the pancreas, and the walls of the small intestines. But enzymes are active in all metabolic processes, providing heat and energy, and building new cells and tissues. In short, enzymes control the cell's chemical reactions. And they are in every cell, including sperm.

There are hundreds of kinds of enzymes, for each enzyme can produce only one kind of reaction. In fact, 2,000 or more enzyme reactions can take place in a single cell. Without the help of enzymes, nutritive substances could not be sufficiently absorbed, nor could metabolic processes be carried out fast enough.

Yet it was not until 1926 that enzymes were isolated, 1940 when they were linked to genes, and 1956 when the DNA in them was proven to be the material of heredity. And by the way, in 1974 a Nobel prize was given to three scientists for their work on methods of dissecting the cell.

An enzyme consists of two parts. The main part doesn't change, but the other part, the coenzyme, breaks off or is used up, and it has to be replaced. The large part is always protein. The coenzyme may be protein or mineral, but very likely it is a vitamin, a protein vitamin. So now we see where vitamins fit in the life process. They work as coenzymes, attaching themselves to specific proteins. But more about vitamins later.

And It All Starts with the Sun's Rays

Such are the cell's most important structures. How marvelous they are, and their ways of working almost unbelievable! And to think it all starts with the sun's rays acting on chlorophyll molecules in green plants. In that action, called photosynthesis, some solar energy becomes electrical energy, but solar energy also causes a chemical reaction that turns carbon dioxide, water and air into carbohydrates, especially into glucose.

Animals eat plants, and in animals each molecule of energy-containing glucose is chemically acted on by ATP (adenosine triphosphate) and a special enzyme to produce pyruvic acid. Both ATP and the enzyme are needed. Then the pyruvic acid molecule is taken up by a mitochondrion in the cell and put through the Krebs citric acid cycle.

The result is that for each pyruvic acid molecule there are now 36 ATP molecules, a great energy gain. Moreover, in each mitochondrion the electric currents move along on electron-transport chains, with the current matched to the need, maybe 30 electrons per second.

In a single mitochondrion there may be 15,000 chains, and in each cell 50-5,000 mitochondria. Then, remember, a single cell may be capable of 2,000 enzyme reactions. Isn't it amazing?

Cells Vary in Function

In spite of their common basic structure, cells can be classed as skin, bone, connective tissue, muscle, nerve, or blood. And they vary within their class. For example, a single nerve cell can be three feet long.

Cells vary also in life span. The epithelial cells of the small intestine can be sloughed off in 1½ days. White blood cells live about two weeks, red blood cells about 4 months, liver cells an estimated 18 months, whereas nerve cells, which normally are not replaced, can live over 100 years. Nor can muscle cells ordinarily be replaced. So it is that 30 percent of muscle cells can be lost between ages 30 and 75. Yet the muscle cells that are left can be made larger and stronger. And in case of accidental damage they can grow back in 9-12 months, nerve cells somewhat longer.

Though red blood cells do not have chromosomes and so cannot reproduce themselves, new blood cells are being made, most in the bone marrow, others in the thymus. Actually it is hemocytoblasts in the bone marrow that become blood cells, most being erythrocytes (*erythros*, red) and some leucocytes (*leukos*, white). The blood cells that come from bone marrow are called B-cells, those from the thymus, T-cells. Still other white blood cells come from the lymph and are called lymphocytes.

Besides transporting nourishment, the main work of the red blood cells is respiration. They carry oxygen from the lungs to the various tissues and then carry back to the lungs the carbon dioxide, which is expelled to feed plant life. So important are the red blood cells that there are about 4-6 million per cu. mm. of blood, including plasma. The white blood cells number only about 4-9 thousand per cu. mm. of blood. But they, too, are essential. The immune system depends on them. In fact, you might say that they are the main part of the immune system.

White Blood Cells and the Immune System

When a virus or harmful bacterium gains entry through mucous linings (and they are doing it all the time), our white blood cells, in fact our whole immune system, goes to work to protect us. So it is that many kinds of cells, including B-cells, T-cells, and fibroblasts (connective tissue cells) produce interferon. That is one of the more recently discovered antibodies.

Interferon acts on many viruses. But it is in short supply, seemingly designed mainly to give time for other antibodies—the lymphocytes and the phagocytes—to get organized.

With the lymph channels concentrated in likely places of infection or of invasion by bacteria, the lymphocytes wall off the infected area, or if need be a dam is made in one of the lymph nodes so as to control the flow of toxic material, something you can feel when the lymph nodes in the throat are swollen.

The lymphocytes also make protein antibodies on a large scale. These attach themselves to the invaders and chemically change them so that they are vulnerable to the phagocytes (*phagein*, eat) which engulf them.

Some phagocytes circulate; others are stationed in the lining of various organs. That's important, for on a second attack by the same invader, the body is immune to it. One phagocyte cell that I can't pass up is the macrophage; it may break up worn-out red blood cells, but then it economically saves the iron for reuse. Since macrophages are connective tissue cells, they are practically everywhere, and as their name implies they are large.

Besides all of the above protective actions taken by the cells, there are other antibodies in the blood—the liver-produced gamma globulines. These, too, attack the invaders and make them harmless.

The Problem of Deterioration

Not only are cells busy taking in food, using it for their special life processes, and protecting themselves from harmful toxins, they also have to contend with their own deterioration. With so many cells being sloughed off, there may be slight changes in the pattern for the new ones, or perhaps the replacement material is inferior or inadequate.

After all, the cells can only take from the blood the nourishment that it carries. And thus they, and we, age and die. That's a necessary process, one that philosophers and scientists have long considered, and now some scientists talk of overcoming. That's not my concern.

Still it is interesting that different mammals have specific life spans. Man's is the longest, and though the *maximum* has long remained practically constant, the average since 1900 has increased 25 years, due especially to the reduction in infant and childhood mortality and to the use of antibiotics.

So though the prospects for longer life at the age of 60 have increased only slightly, more people are reaching that age. Certainly today's knowledge permits us to live more healthfully, and there can be no question as to the value of laboratory studies of nutrition and longevity.

What about the "Free Radicals"?

Regarding the various theories of aging, it is said, "the free radical theory, the crosslinking theory, the decline of neurotransmitters, and the biological clock theory all involve free radicals." (Durk Pearson and Sandy Shaw, *Life Extension*, 1982, p. 153)

In case you are not familiar with this use of the word *radical*, here's how the dictionary puts it: a radical is an "atom or a group of atoms acting as a unit in chemical reactions." For example, ammonium (NH_4) is a radical in NH_4Cl. And a free radical is an atom or group of atoms having at least one unpaired electron. Free radicals are in all living systems, being produced from air, water, food, radiation, etc. Some are necessary for metabolism, others cause much trouble. It's the latter that we hear so much about.

Likewise with the term *oxidation*, it can be good or bad. It replaced the broader term *combustion*, because it is more descriptive of how the cells of the body transform their food into energy. Oxygen makes up 65 percent of all the chemical elements in the human body, carbon 18.5, hydrogen 9.5, nitrogen 3.3, calcium 1.5, and the other elements even less. A cell's life depends on oxidation, yet oxygen is so strong that it needs to work in combination, as in water, H_2O. Trouble arises when there is too much oxygen. That, it seems, should be described as peroxidation, *per* meaning maximum or too much. But *oxidation* is the term used, and it usually refers to too much. So we need antioxidants.

Even crosslinking of an atom usually refers to a negative reaction, though there are those that do no damage.

Help through Free-radical Scavengers and Antioxidants

Now consider the case of oxygen interacting with polyunsaturated lipids (fats). That produces free radicals. Then, on the one hand, these free radicals cause the failure of the T-cells to provide immunity and so cause infectious diseases, atherosclerosis, even cancer; while on the other hand, such peroxided lipids may inhibit the hormone that prevents the formation of abnormal blood clots, and thus perhaps cause a stroke.

Then, too, free radicals can interfere with protein synthesis, with the result that cross-linking both of collagen and of muscle atoms results in deterioration in those systems, causing stiffening and loss of elasticity. Free radicals also cross-link with the cell's DNA, which carries the very pattern of the cell's continuing life.

What can the cells do about free radicals, oxidation, and cross-linking? Says Saul Kent in *The Life Extension Revolution*, 1980, p. 127, "There is a battery of enzymes—including catalases, peroxidases, and superoxide dismutases—that protect cells against oxygen toxicity by serving as free-radical scavengers." And he further points to the protection against oxidative attack that can be obtained from antioxidants.

Quite likely you are familiar with some of the antioxidants, especially the fat-soluble vitamins A, D, E, and K. These can pass into the cells only if attached to a molecule of fat, but they can be stored in the body, especially in the liver. Besides these, Pearson and Shaw's list of antioxidants includes B_1, B_5, B_6, the amino acid cysteine, the food preservatives BHT and BHA, and the minerals zinc and selenium.

In Part II we have seen how the body gets nourished and how it takes care of itself, so now we should be better able to consider its needs and how to meet them.

I ADORE THEE THIS MOMENT

The bloom of thine cheek, which was tinted with red
  Like the roses of summer, has faded and gone;
Thine eyes have grown dim, their bright sparkle has fled
  With the years that have fleeted so rapidly on
Since that ju-bi-lant day when we gayly were wed.
  Yet dearer and sweeter, charm that thou art,
Is thyself, which is brighter than ever before:
  Whilst I loved thee in youth from the depth of my heart,
I adore thee this moment and love thee still more!

Dad (Robert H. Pallister)

PART III

PUTTING THINGS IN PERSPECTIVE

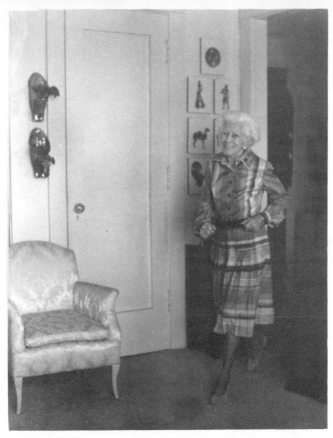

Running, in my apartment,   May, 1984

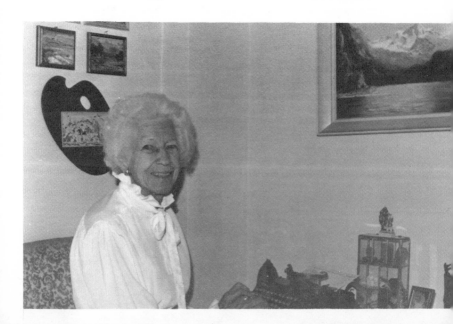

Vitamins—Their Natural Sources

Certainly, the body needs vitamins. As you will remember, vitamins work by joining enzymes. These then spark the body's digestive and metabolic processes, which otherwise would be too slow.

By definition vitamins are organic substances that are required for the growth and nourishment of the body that are found in small amounts in plant and animal foods. It was not until 1911 that the term vitamin (then spelled vitamine) was used to describe C as the agent in rice polish that would prevent beriberi. Since then one vitamin after another has been isolated in foods, and now many are manufactured.

A list of vitamins with their food sources, also their synthetic forms, is given in *Nutrition Almanac*, John Kirschmann, Dir., 1979, pp. 102-4. It gives yeast as the natural source for B_1, B_2, B_3, B_5, B_6, B_{12}, biotin, folic acid, and PABA. Then for choline and inositol, soybeans are the first source, yeast the second.

Apricot kernels are given as the natural source for B_{17}, (laetrile) and B_{15} (pangamic acid). For C, it is rose hips, acerola berries, and others; for D, codliver oil; for E, vegetable oils; for F, unsaturated fatty acids (vegetable oils); for K, alfalfa; and for bioflavonoids, rutin, hesperin and others.

Vitamins are not concentrated bits of food that can be digested to nourish the body. Rather, vitamins are certain minute parts of food that serve as coenzymes and so spark the physiological processes of life, and which the body has to have supplied in or with its food. Moreover, the amounts needed vary from one individual to another and for the same person in different conditions of health.

Vitamins are readily classified as water-soluble and fat-soluble. The B vitamins and C are water-soluble; A, D, E, and K are fat-soluble. For the most part the B's and C are not stored, and any excess is excreted. The fat-soluble vitamins can be stored, and if taken in excess over a long period of time can be harmful.

Minerals—The Body Can't Make Any

Important as vitamins are, minerals also are essential to the life process. In fact, the balance of the potassium within the cell with the sodium in the fluid surrounding it is critical to the cell's nourishment, for it is their action that draws chemical substances in and out of the cell, for example, food in, waste out. Not enough potassium and the cells become waterlogged; not enough sodium and they lose nourishment.

Unlike vitamins, minerals form constituent parts of the body, especially as seen in bones and teeth. Like vitamins, minerals act as coenzymes. In fact, most vitamins can't work without minerals. Minerals are both alkalizing and acid-forming, and they keep the body from becoming too acid or too alkaline. Moreover, minerals carry electrical charges, and nerve impulses are dependent on minerals.

The body can't make a single mineral. They're inorganic, and in general are plentiful in water and soil. We get them in natural plant and animal foods as well as in water. For example, brewer's yeast has 14 minerals; kelp also is rich in minerals. As with vitamins, individual mineral requirements differ. Yet a table of minerals, classified by Abram Hoffer and Morton Walker as to quantity, puts the estimated daily requirements in perspective.

Estimated Daily Requirements of Minerals

In grams		In mg.		Less than 1 mg.
Sodium	5	Iron	15	Molybdenum
Potassium	4	Zinc	15	Cobalt
Phosphorus	2	Manganese	5	Selenium
Calcium	1	Copper	2	Lithium
Magnesium	.35	Chromium	2	Iodine

From *Orthomolecular Nutrition*, Keats Publishing, Inc., 1978, p. 150. Credit for estimated amounts given to R. J. Williams and Carl C. Peiffer.

Not surprisingly, sodium and potassium are highest in the amount needed daily by the human body. Fortunately they are widespread in natural foods. Yet, plentiful as minerals are, there are deficiencies, due to different individual requirements and to the fact that in general the assimilation of minerals is not easy. For example, it is found that calcium is only 20-40 percent absorbed, iron even less.

So it is that chelated minerals are recommended. In the normal process of digestion, minerals are bonded with amino acids, that is, if there is a suitable amino acid available. To avoid taking that chance, mineral supplements can be bought already chelated.

Another point about minerals is that they form part of gland secretions.

Hormones—They're Potent Too

The endocrine glands and their secretions make yet another system that influences body functions. As with enzymes, vitamins, and minerals, hormones act and interact throughout the body.

In fact, it is said, "Hormones, even in extremely tiny amounts, are unbelievably potent; they direct and regulate much of the subtle biochemistry of life." (Henry G. Bieler, M.D., *Food Is Your Best Medicine*, 1965, p. 70) Bieler then goes on to explain how the adrenal glands control the oxidation of all body cells, the tone of muscles, the number of circulating blood cells, the degree of their immunity, and more.

Likewise, other glands secrete different hormones with specific functions. Then the blood going through the glands picks up the hormones and carries them to the part of the body that they are intended to stimulate, slow down, or change. That's the way the various glands work: the pituitary, the thyroid, the thymus, the liver, the kidneys, and the rest, but the pancreas, as already noted, also has a duct. How well the glands function depends on how they are nourished and kept free of toxins.

In the glands and everywhere, the cells take from the blood stream the nutrients they need and can get. Always they strive to live, some with better chances than others. They are so dependent on the nourishment they are given. Though it is true that the body can synthesize some vitamins and some amino acids and it makes its hormones, still all of its nourishment actually comes from the food we give it.

But what are its proper nutrients?

The Body's Nutrient Composition

"By supplying our body daily with the elements of which it is composed, we can have complete health, provided we give due thought, attention, and consideration to the other two parts of our being, namely, our Mind and our Spirit." So says N. W. Walker in *Fresh Vegetable and Fruit Juices*, 1978, p. 9. And Dr. Walker is the one nutritionist over 100 years old.

So let's consider the body's nutrient composition. Did you know it's about two thirds water? Here are some figures.

Nutrient Composition of the Body in Percent

		Solids only
Water	67	
Proteins	15	45.5
Fats	13	39.4
Minerals	4	12.1
Carbohydrates	1	3.0
	100	100.0

From Louis Levine, *Biology for a Modern Society*, 1977, p. 23.

If it seems surprising that carbohydrates are so low, bear in mind that their storage capacity is small. In fact, their depots are exhausted after 24 hours without food. So carbohydrates need daily replacement, for they are our chief source of energy, 50 percent. Fats furnish 40 percent. Protein is used when the other two are insufficient. In that case the body will convert up to 58 percent of one's daily protein intake to sugar for fuel. Yet, though protein can substitute for carbohydrates and fats, neither carbohydrates nor fats can do the work of proteins.

It's proteins that do the actual work in the cells. There each chemical reaction is catalyzed by a specific protein in an enzyme. In fact, it is said that humans have about 50,000 different proteins. Not only are proteins the stuff of enzymes, but also of antibodies in the cell's immune system and of gamma globulins. Collagen, the protein substance in the fiber of connective tissue, is 40 percent of the body's protein. Even hair is protein. No wonder proteins are called the building blocks of the body.

Fats, furnishing twice the calories of either carbohydrates or proteins, are recognized for their role in energy production, but if absent the body converts carbohydrates to fats, for fats are also needed to transport and absorb the fat-soluble vitamins, namely, the antioxidants. Then, too, fats are needed for gallbladder action.

Fat also provides support for the various organs. When more is supplied than is needed, it is stored as energy reserves. But of course one can take in too much fat, which then slows digestion and metabolism and causes trouble.

We need both the saturated and the unsaturated fats—the solids and the oils. In fact, there are three unsaturated ones (already given on p. 24) that the body cannot synthesize. However, if one of them, linoleic, is supplied, then the body can make the other two if the necessary vitamins and minerals are provided. Linoleic acid's best sources are safflower, sunflower-seed, walnut and soy oils.

Cholesterol, a fat-related substance, is a constituent of most cells, especially those of the brain and nervous system, the liver, and blood. But when it was found in plaque deposits on the walls of arteries, it was blamed for arteriosclerosis. However, cutting down on the consumption of foods containing cholesterol did not help, for the body simply made more. Moreover, "Studies have shown that approximately 800 milligrams of cholesterol are obtained daily from a high-fat diet, whereas a normal adult liver produces 3,000 milligrams or more per day." (Adelle Davis, *Let's Eat Right to Keep Fit*, 1954, p. 41)

Cholesterol is a needed nutrient made in the liver and intestine and furnished healthfully in such foods as eggs; in fact, lecithin, onions, garlic, eggplant, as well as eggs, carry in them a factor that breaks up cholesterol, so that it goes through blood vessels without clogging them.

The important thing to remember about fats, then, is to provide them with the substances that prevent clogged arteries and the accumulation of too much fat in the liver.

Oils are frequently harmed by being hydrogenated, that is, having hydrogen forced through them to harden them or by being highly heated, as in deep frying. Both Adelle Davis and Gladys Lindberg advise against these two practices, and I have pretty much followed these nutritionists in that.

So far, I have pointed to the importance of carbohydrates, but they, too, can be harmful, especially sucrose, the consumption of which is extremely high in this country—about 125 pounds of sugar a year for every man, woman and child. That includes processed foods, so we are not likely aware of it.

Yet through the ages our digestive system got no sugar at all as we know it. No wonder it cannot handle so much now. In trying to maintain the proper glucose level by the insulin hormone, as is natural, too much sugar either produces too much insulin, which lowers the sugar content of the blood, or it so damages the pancreas that it can no longer produce enough insulin.

The harm of too much sugar in the diet makes a long story, which includes not only obesity and its resulting ills but also atherosclerosis and more. I'll mention further only the effect on disposition. Says Adelle Davis, "The person whose blood sugar falls below normal becomes progressively more irritable, grouchy, moody, depressed, and unco-operative." (*Let's Eat Right to Keep Fit*, 1954, p. 10)

After commenting on how common low blood sugar is today, Dr. Harold Rosenberg remarks, "Certainly a general grouchiness and irritability seem a current and unwelcome aspect of American life. . . . Very little of a spirit of good-natured tolerance and compromise is in evidence." (*The Book of Vitamin Therapy*, 1974, p. 128)

Minerals were discussed earlier, as their function with enzymes is so important, and it was stated that they are body constituents. In the body's composition, minerals represent about a third the weight of fats, a fourth that of proteins; in short, they are four percent of the total, whereas water is 67 percent.

We've seen how the body reuses water; still that excreted has to be replaced. Eight glasses a day is commonly recommended, but I find that too much for me. Gladys Lindberg recommends six—one before each meal and one immediately after.

The big question is the kind of water—tap, distilled, or untreated. I use tap, though I'd prefer spring water, but the delivered quantity is too great and lugging it in is too difficult. So I often use vegetable and fruit juices. Henry Bieler, M.D., calls the water in such juices "natural water," and Norman Walker, D.Sc., says, "The reason for the efficacy of such juices lies in the fact that, by separating the mineral elements and the distilled water in the food from the fibers, this liquid food is digested in a matter of minutes." (*Fresh Vegetable and Fruit Juices*, 1978, p. 5)

What's Needed for Replacement?

That's the telling question, and it is a complicated one. Since 1943 the Food and Nutrition Board of the National Research Council of the National Academy of Science has been issuing standards or recommendations. Here's how the 1980 report opens:

"Recommended Dietary Allowances (RDA) are the levels of intake of essential nutrients considered, in the judgment of the Committee on Dietary Allowances of the Food and Nutrition Board on the basis of available scientific knowledge, to be adequate to meet the known nutritional needs of practically all healthy persons."

After that heading, the opening sentence says: "RDA are recommended for the daily amounts of nutrients that *population groups* should consume over a period of time." (p. 1) And further, "The requirement for a nutrient is the minimum intake that will maintain normal function and health." (p. 3)

Then, too, "Following a review of scientific evidence of nutritional requirements judged by the Committee on Dietary Allowances to be most reliable, a logical approach in setting recommended allowances for nutrients other than energy is to select a value above the average requirement by an amount that includes the range of variability observed." (p. 3-4)

The important thing to note, it seems, is that the RDA are based on data of the nutritional dietary intake of "apparently normal healthy people." The stated aim is to maintain good health, not to reach the optimum, nor of course to cover those not in good health. Moreover, the RDA are judgments of the group of scientists.

RECOMMENDED DIETARY ALLOWANCES

A comparison of RDA (Food and Nutrition Board), My average, and Supplements

Item and measure used	RDA women 51-	My average (2 days)	* Kenyon's Super Nutrients	* Lindberg's Formula (p. 182)	* Rosenberg's Women 60- (p. 167)
1 Calories	1850	1408			
2 Carbohydrates (grams)	277	166			
3 Proteins (grams)	46	56			
4 Fats (grams)	59	60			
5 A (International Units)	4000	41,000	25,000	25,000	20,000-30,000
6 D "	400		400	400	800-1200
7 B_1 (Thiamine) mg.	1.0	2.9	200.0	20.0	200-300
8 B_2 (Riboflavin) mg.	1.2	3.3	20.0	30.0	150-300
9 B_3 (Niacin) mg.	13.0	19.6	100	100	400-2000
10 B_5 (Pantothenic acid) mg.	-10	8.4	250	100	100-200
11 B_6 (Pyridoxine) mg.	2.0	2.3	200	20	200-600
12 B_{12} (mcg.)	3.0	38.1	200	25	50-100
13 Biotin (mcg.)	150-300	169	25	25	300-600
14 Folic Acid (mg.)	0.4	0.6	0.1	0.4	2-5
15 C (mg.)	45	151	2500	500	1000-5000
16 E (IU)	12	17.7	500	200	600-800

17	Sodium (mg.)	1100-3300	1437	—	—	—
18	Phosphorus (mg.)	800	1889	75	—	1000-2000
19	Potassium (mg.)	1875-5625	3936	99	25	—
20	Calcium (mg.)	800	1950	200	400	1000-2000
21	Iron (mg.)	10	16.6	10	18	20-60
22	Magnesium (mg.)	300	940	100	200	400-800
23	Copper (mg.)	2-3	3	0.25	1	2-4
24	Manganese (mg.)	2.5-5	2.3	10	5	—
25	Selenium (mg.)	.05-.2	0.07	0.2	0.05	—
26	Zinc (mg.)	15	5.1	25	30	15-30
27	Iodine (mcg.)	0.225		0.225	0.15	.15-.30
28	Chromium (mcg.)			20	50	—
29	Choline (mg.)	500-900		500	100	250-1000
30	Inositol (mg.)			20	100	1000
31	PABA (mg.)			500	50	200
32	Cysteine (mg.)			850		
33	Methionine (mg.)			200		

*Data used by permission
Keith Kenyon, M.D. From container.
Gladys Lindberg and Judy Lindberg McFarland, *Take Charge of Your Health*, Harper & Row, c. 1982.
Dr. Harold Rosenberg & A. N. Feldzamen, PhD, G. P. Putnam's Sons, *The Book of Vitamin Therapy*, c. 1974.

A Comparison with the RDA

Even with the data thus limited, I wondered how my "intake" would compare with the RDA. To find out was quite a bit of work, but I do recommend that you do the same. Until you do, I trust the analysis of these data on pages 60-61 will give you a better appreciation of the importance of your daily intake.

My procedure was to average my intake of two days (col. 2) and then compare it with the RDA (col. 1). I used the Food Composition tables in *Nutrition Almanac*, 4th ed., John D. Kirschmann, director, 1979, though there are others. What I found was that my intake is surprisingly close to the RDA, the notable differences being explainable or acceptable. Although my calorie intake (line 1) appears low by this table, another table that goes down to my height and weight puts the calorie figure for me at 1249, and my record is well above that. (David Rubincam and John Rubincam, *Diet the Natural Way*, 1977, p. 119)

As for the carbohydrates (line 2), a similar correction for weight fails to bring my carbohydrate intake up to the RDA, but if I then added just five dates I'd be near enough. And I might say that many people probably get those extra carbohydrate grams by having a piece of gingerbread for lunch and a piece of apple pie for dinner.

My protein intake (line 3) is high according to the RDA, but not according to Adelle Davis, and with the Lindberg recommendation of adding 10 grams of protein to the RDA "as a safety margin," it seems not too bad. (*Take Charge of Your Health*, 1982, p. 67)

With all our body's facilities for handling protein, I see no need for concern. Not only do protein foods appeal to our taste buds, but except for water, protein is the body's biggest component.

Further Analysis of Differences

Regarding the vitamins (lines 5-16, 29-31), the most marked difference between my diet and the RDA is that I get much more vitamin A, due mainly to having a cup of carrot juice (24,750 IU) one day, and the other day, liver (37,400 IU). Although A is stored in the body and too much can be toxic, it has to be in much greater amounts and continued over a long period. B_{12} also was high, due to three ounces of liver having 68 mcg. of it.

Of the minerals (lines 17-28), the phosphorus and calcium balance, as is proper, but it was hard to tell about the sodium and potassium. Both are within the acceptable range, yet I do think I've been too sparing of salt. It is true that for a person with high blood pressure, decreasing the salt intake lowers the pressure. But mine is already low (130 over 74), which is said to favor long life. On the other hand, "People with adrenaline exhaustion usually have low blood pressure, which indicates that salt should be obtained." (Adelle Davis, *Let's Get Well*, p. 294) Davis also says it might be better for some people with high blood pressure to increase their potassium rather than reduce their sodium.

The other mineral intakes appear normal except for zinc. However, my table gave no amounts of zinc in yeast, soy, or eggs, yet those items are given as high sources of that mineral.

It is interesting that Canada, Japan, and the World Health Organization also give tables of RDA. Though there are differences, the four are much alike, especially if compared with a megavitamin table. See Rosenberg, Column 5.

Rightly or wrongly, I conclude that my dietary intake is not much out of line with the RDA. Anyhow here is what I ate those two days. For breakfast both days I had my mix (see p. 25) plus one half a peach one day and one half an apple the other.

Then for one day the midday meal included one cup of carrot juice, sardines, rice, broccoli, a gherkin, and one half a cup of sliced cucumber. The other meal consisted of one large egg, a slice of whole-wheat bread, cheese, and a medium tomato.

On the other day I had a cup of buttermilk, liver, baked potato, butter, string beans, one-half cup of alfalfa sprouts with Thousand Island dressing; and for supper a slice of whole-wheat bread, one half avocado, one cup of vegetable-juice cocktail, and one eighth cup of raisins.

Both days' intake included an evening snack of a banana. That, I really look forward to. Sometimes I have a snack during the day, perhaps a glass of raw milk and peanut butter on a cracker, especially if I'm not having milk at a meal.

I try to have buttermilk with liver, because liver is high in cholesterol, and buttermilk carries lecithin, which breaks up the cholesterol so that it doesn't form plaque. The rest of the story is that in making butter, the milk's lecithin goes into the buttermilk and its cholesterol into the butter. (Linda Clark, *Stay Young Longer*, 1961, p. 165)

A head of lettuce is a lot for a person alone, so I use alfalfa sprouts, which, by the way, are helpful for the "floating" test. I don't use bran.

The Amino Acids

I did wonder also about the amino acids, for increasingly one reads about this or that amino acid. Now amino acids are simply the components of protein, and there are 22 of general application. Eight of them are called "essential."

In the table on page 66 you'll see the Estimated Amino Acid Requirement (EAAR) for these essential amino acids per kilogram of one's weight and for a 90-pound person; also the amounts in a few foods.

With a normal intake of varied proteins, the essential amino acids are probably provided satisfactorily; vegetarians, however, need to check. And in spite of the likely coverage of the essential amino acids, there are points that should be noted.

First, amino acids have co-factors, namely, vitamins and minerals. If they are missing, there won't be enzymes to work on the amino acids so that they can be used for making body protein.

Then, too, amino acids are useful only in amounts and proportions that approximate the body's requirements. Thus, in any protein food there is a limiting amino acid (LAA), the one that provides the lowest percent of the estimated daily amino acid requirement.

In the foods listed, in fact, in most foods, methionine is the limiting amino acid. Yet it is broadly needed, having many functions: Methionine increases the liver's production of lecithin. It provides sulfur, deactivates free radicals, chelates heavy metals, and it is necessary for the production of cysteine, an amino acid in the sulfur-containing group with methionine.

Cysteine, too, deactivates free radicals, acts as an antioxidant, and so aids the immune system. And note this: "One egg supplies approximately 65 mg. of sulfur and one gram of the amino acid cysteine, which as cysteine hydrochloride supplies approximately 180 mg. of sulfur." So says Robert

ESSENTIAL AMINO ACIDS (in mgs.)

Essential Amino Acids	Req'd per kg. of wt.	For 90-pound person	Whole wheat bread 1 slice	Egg 1 med. size	Butter-milk 1 cup	Tuna fish 3 oz.	Squash seeds ¼ cup	Broc-coli 1 cup
Isoleucine	12	452	106	420	514	1253	934	157
Leucine	16	656	166	559	809	1850	1309	202
Lysine	12	452	71	406	678	2155	767	181
Methionine	10	410	37	197	188	710	317	61
Phenylalanine	16	656	117	369	433	303	934	149
Threonine	8	328	72	318	384	1254	500	153
Tryptophan	3	123	29	102	90	245	300	45
Valine	14	574	113	470	613	1303	900	210

Requirements per kilogram of weight from National Academy of Sciences, *Recommended Dietary Allowances*, 1980, p. 43.
Values for foods from *Nutrition Almanac*, John D. Kirschmann, Director, 1979, pp. 237-43.

Garrison in *Lysine, Tryptophan, and Other Amino Acids*, 1982, p. 14.

Tryptophan's rather newly heralded service is that it acts as a precursor for serotin, an inhibitory neurotransmitter required for sleep. However, tryptophan won't act as a sleeping pill if it closely follows a high protein meal or snack, for then other amino acids bar it from getting to the brain. Tryptophan has also been found helpful for lessening depression and in building immunity.

Both cysteine and tryptophan are used by Pearson and Shaw in their experimental formula, as is also arginine, a nonessential amino acid. (*Life Extension*, 1982, pp. 468-9)

No doubt there are conditions that can be helped by a given amino acid. But meat, fish, poultry, and dairy products provide complete amino acids, and when accompanied by a raw vegetable or fruit (for their vitamins and minerals), these protein foods generally take care of our amino acid needs.

As for methionine, most fish supply somewhat more of this limiting essential amino acid than do meats, poultry, or dairy products. Especially do tuna, flounder, and swordfish stand high in methionine.

The Matter of Supplements

Wisely or foolishly, I take extra vitamins for insurance, and have for the last 15-20 years, including the formulas given in the table on pages 60-61. And I have added to them considerably more C, E, B_3, and if not included, digestive enzymes and bioflavonoids. For comparison, this table also includes the RDA of the Food and Nutrition Board and Dr. Rosenberg's higher amounts. He is a practicing physician and past president of the International Academy of Preventive Medicine, and has used vitamins as therapy for his patients.

Although a great many research studies have been made to determine deficiency states and their effects, and much has been learned from them about the body's need for the different vitamins and minerals, little has been learned about the optimums except in the course of practice by physicians with individual patients.

So it is that two schools of thought have developed. One group of professionals holds that there is no need for extra vitamins. (Remember, my diet met the Food and Nutrition Board's RDA.) Says Louis Levine, "Unfortunately, the vitamin supplements available provide far greater amounts of vitamins than an individual can conceivably need." (*Biology for a Modern Society*, 1977, p. 64) And he goes on to say it's a tremendous economic waste.

Other competent professionals recommend mega-supplements. Richard Kunin says, "Linus Pauling has given the rationale: The greater the concentration of molecules in a chemical reaction, the faster the reaction will proceed." (*Mega Nutrition*, 1980, p. 244)

My diet appears to give the Recommended Dietary Allowances. Moreover, since the amounts of vitamins in the body are minimal, and since natural foods tend to furnish them in proper proportion, and since some can be synthesized, and since I anyhow play safe with supplements of vitamins and minerals, it seems I hardly need worry.

Of course I'm not making any recommendations. Diets and supplements are very much an individual matter. Just thought you might be curious.

Extra Vitamin C

Although supplements are very much an individual matter, I do want to comment on vitamin C. Many people think that they are getting enough C in a multiple vitamin, but usually it is only 200-500 mg. Yet vitamin C is neither made nor stored by our body, and we need an ample and constant supply.

Vitamin C plays a part in the basic metabolic process of life in every cell. And it helps make collagen, the protein substance that holds the cells together. With calcium, it gives collagen its strength. On the other hand, a deficiency of C causes the capillaries to become fragile and appears to increase cholesterol, thus leading to atherosclerosis.

Vitamin C works better with other vitamins, especially vitamin P, a bioflavonoid which increases capillary strength. Moreover, vitamin C appears able to function for other vitamins. And it combines with toxins to destroy them. So it is especially effective in fighting infection. If taken early and in sufficient amount, it can usually stop a cold or at least lighten its effect. At least it does for me if I start at the very first sign of a cold and take 1,000 mg. every hour, even into the night, if I wake up.

Old people especially need vitamin C, but they should not think they get enough in a glass of orange juice. It has only 129 mg. in eight ounces. A cup of broccoli has 105 mg, a medium tomato only 35. I regularly take about 4,000 mg. a day.

When vitamin C is taken, it reaches a maximum in the blood in two to three hours. The body of a normal person of average weight contains about 5,000 mg. of C when it is fully saturated. But vitamin C is out of the body in three or four hours. So it is important to keep up your C supply.

Extra Vitamin E

Another vitamin I must give space to is E. It, like C, is said to strengthen capillary walls, also muscles. Especially is it recommended for the heart. Moreover, it decreases blood clotting and improves circulation, that is, by combining with oxygen. On the other hand, oxygen, as already noted, can get out of control and damage cells or make the wrong combinations. In such cases vitamin E, like other antioxidants, prevents or slows down the oxidation. In these ways vitamin E serves as an anticoagulant, a vasodialator, and an antioxidant.

For a time some years ago my lower legs would pain so on walking it was all I could do to walk across a wide street without resting. I started taking vitamin E and got over the trouble, and I have kept on taking extra E, 800 IU (international units) per day.

However, vitamin E is not recommended for people with a rheumatic heart. And those with high blood pressure or diabetes are advised to start with a low amount. With that said, *Earl Mindell's Vitamin Bible* gives 200-1,200 IU as the daily doses most often used.

Another vasodialator is garlic, and I have had many spells of taking it. Now I'm finishing a bottle of garlic and parsley capsules. But I've been taking only two a day instead of two a meal, as Morton Walker recommends in *The Chelation Answer*, 1982. There he lists 14 ways whereby purified garlic helps the body processes, the first being as an antibiotic. (p. 133)

The mineral selenium works with vitamin E to increase its antioxidant effect, but selenium can be toxic, so the usual dosage is only 50-150 mcg., though more is sometimes prescribed as defense against carcinogens.

Extra Vitamin B-3

I would also give special mention to Niacin (B-3). I started taking extra B-3 some time ago, when I first read about Dr. Abram Hoffer giving his mother nicotinic acid, three grams per day, which corrected early signs of senility.

Surely there is nothing that oldsters fear more than becoming senile. So I have been taking one half of what Dr. Hoffer gave his mother, 500 mg. of niacinamide per meal. Niacinamide doesn't cause flushing.

Now I find Dr. Hoffer reporting the circumstances in the case of his mother in *Nutrients to Age Without Senility* by Abram Hoffer and Morton Walker, 1980, and Dr. Hoffer reports that he added vitamins C and E. (p. 11) In the chapter, "The Antisenility Vitamins," pantothenic acid is also included, 250-750 mg. per day. (p. 147)

Earl Mindell's Vitamin Bible lists niacin's benefits (p. 60), then cautions: "Niacin should be used cautiously by anyone with severe diabetes, glaucoma, peptic ulcers, or with impaired liver function." (p. 151)

I find it interesting that Pearson and Shaw talk of niacinamide's tranquilizing effect. They say we have natural brain chemicals that "induce calm and tranquility. The form of B-3 called niacinamide seems to be one such compound." (*Life Extention*, 1982, p. 282) And they go on to suggest that with inosital and GABA, an amino acid, it might substitute for Valium and Librium, at least in part.

Chelation for Unclogging Arteries

Some years ago I looked into chelation therapy, but found the cost would likely be $1500 to $2000. Chelation therapy consists of a series of injections primarily of *ethylene diamine tetraacetic acid* (EDTA), which draws, as by a claw (Latin *chele*, claw) plaque from the walls of arteries.

EDTA was first used for removing lead from the system, but in that process it was found to also help atherosclerosis. Besides lead, it also removes mercury, unwanted calcium and more. This is a great boon to those with atherosclerosis and related ills and especially for those considering by-pass heart surgery.

Now I find in *The Chelation Answer* by Morton Walker, 1982, a chapter entitled "How to Chelate Yourself at Home." It is not offered as a substitute for EDTA chelation therapy, but rather as a preventative.

What especially interests me is that my diet and supplements include all of the recommended substances and, except for garlic, in the range of amounts recommended: C, 4000 mg. plus bioflavonoids; B-3, 50 mg.-3 gr.; B-6, 250 mg.; E, 100-800 IU; DMG (in B-15) 90-270 mg. (in yeast and liver); selenium, 100-200 mcg.; magnesium, 1000 mg. (preferably in aspartate and orotate forms); manganese, 5-25 mg.; bromelain, amount not given, but pineapple is the source; garlic, 270 mg. tablets, 2 each meal; onions, "Something in onions provides a chelating effect." And "high fiber foods are excellent chelating agents." Exercise, too, is given as a chelator. (pp. 120-136)

Then in *Take Charge of Your Health*, 1982, by Gladys Lindberg and Judy Lindberg McFarland, it is said, "Lecithin, inositol, choline, chelated mineral supplements, alfalfa, vitamin C, vitamin E, garlic, rutin, kelp, some legumes, and sulfured amino acids have all been shown to act as chelating agents." (p. 97)

Sardines for Nucleic Acid and More

I think I should mention *Dr. Frank's No Aging Diet* (1976), because it has influenced my diet. Dr. Frank's theory about aging, like others, starts with growth at the cell level with repeated cell division and with each new cell always carrying the original pattern. As time goes on, the pattern somehow gets changed. Theories vary as to how this happens. Frank's is that the genetic code gets damaged in many ways.

What is important is that the DNA, a nucleic acid in the nucleus of every cell, carrying the genetic code and acting on RNA, another nucleic acid in the cell, can be influenced by foods high in nucleic acid. The sardine is one of those foods.

Dr. Frank is not the only one to praise the sardine. In *Dr. Cantor's Longevity Diet* (1967) it is said that there is a widespread deficiency of vanadium and zinc and that these minerals are in sardines, which also reduce cholesterol. In fact, Dr. Cantor, (Alfred J.) says that fish is the answer for longevity.

Then in *Vitality and Aging* (1981) Drs. James F. Fries and Lawrence M. Crapo say that aging is not due to senescence genes, but to errors in the translation of DNA into protein. (p. 40)

If nucleic acid came in a powder, I might put it in my breakfast mix. As things are, I now eat more sardines (drained). And I try to get plenty of water for them to swim in, as is cautioned.

So, who knows, maybe I'll yet pass the "pinch" test. It shows the elasticity of the skin. Just pinch the skin on the back of your hand and watch it go back to normal. I have not had a good score on that for some time. But on the "squeeze the ankle" test, I'm ok.

That brings me to a point I want to be sure to make.

Most Important: Expect to Feel Good Again and Again

My feeling so good is not 100 percent of the time. There are poor days, and I've had enough of them to make me recognize them as "just one of those days." The point I want to make is that at first I was surprised to again feel so good; now I expect it.

Then, too, I've found that though I start out real spry, I may come home quite fatigued. But this also passes when I give the body its proper rest. It's a hard lesson to learn, for we judge by past experience and then have to learn that we don't have the energy we used to have.

Another thing my years have taught me comes from seeing friends terribly sick come back to good health. The body has amazing recuperative powers. One should never give up. Expect the good, and lo and behold, it comes.

Maybe I'm an optimist, but what's wrong with that? Back in the second century Marcus Aurelius said, "Our life is what our thoughts make it." Now it's said, "Only you can make yourself happy." (Janet Rainwater, *You're in Charge*, 1979, p. 197)

Moreover, modern science can demonstrate thought power by the technique of bio-feedback, whereby one can raise or lower his body temperature and effect many other measurable body changes. Indeed, thinking has been shown to change body chemistry.

On the other hand, improved body chemistry is reflected in a brighter mental outlook. As already mentioned (p. 57), low blood sugar can cause one to be depressed. Then, too, deficiency studies of several vitamins have shown that depression can come from a deficiency of vitamins B_1, B_3, B_5, B_6, C, or E, especially B_3 (niacin), and also from a deficiency of certain minerals, especially magnesium, calcium, or zinc.

Primarily these substances work by improving metabolism —giving us more energy, better digestion, and improved nerve action. Certainly the better the body functions, the better one feels, the happier one is.

Then, too, specific substances work on specific organs. For example, vitamin C was discovered by its help in curing scurvy, and B$_3$ (niacin) for its use in curing pellagra, which is notable for its inflammation and peeling of the skin. Then there are the minerals, iodine for preventing goiter, and calcium and magnesium for preventing softening of the bones.

So it works both ways. Our health affects our attitudes. Our attitudes affect our health. And we ourselves can improve both. In a study of longevity among some Indians in Ecuador, the author says, "The Viejos (old ones) were happy, and perhaps that is success in living." (Grace Halsell, *Los Viejos*, 1976, p. 108)

And I like Ella Wilcox's saying: "The truest greatness lies in being kind, the truest wisdom in a happy mind." Yes, I want to be happy, but I want you to be happy, too. So I hope something herein will help you to travel along healthfully and happily to fourscore and ten, and more.

Perhaps this little prayer will assist you, as it does me, in putting things in perspective.

Lord, I have time, I have plenty of time,
All the time that you give me,
The years of my life, The days of my years,
The hours of my days, They are all mine.
Mine to fill, quietly, calmly,
But to fill completely, up to the brim,
To offer them to you, that of their insipid water
You may make a rich wine such as you made once in Cana
    of Galilee.
I am not asking you today, Lord, for time to do this and then
    that,
But your grace to do conscientiously, in the time that you
    give me, what you want me to do.

                        from "Prayers" by Michael Quoist